AIR FRYER REVOLUTION

Your Everyday Air Fryer Book

With Quick & Easy Recipes for Beginners

KetonUSA

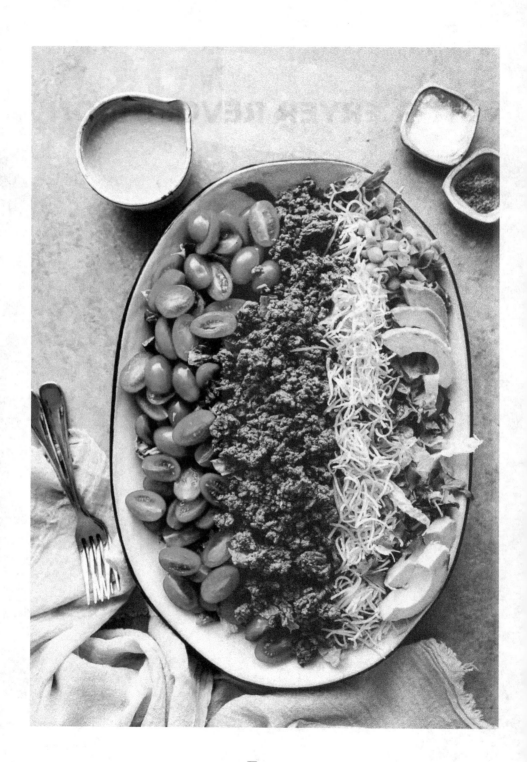

Table of Contents

Pork Rind Tortillas

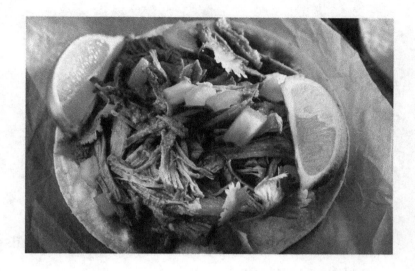

You won't believe how low-carb these Pork Rind Tortillas are! There's no need to buy low-carb tortillas at the store, which are usually made with wheat flour. With just a few simple ingredients, you'll have the perfect gluten-free base for tacos, burritos, or even chips!

- **Hands On Time:** 10 minutes

- **Cook Time:** 5 minutes

Ingredients:

4 tortillas (1 per serving)

- 1 ounce pork rinds

- 3/4 cup shredded mozzarella cheese

- 2 tablespoons full-fat cream cheese

- 1 large egg

Directions

1. Place pork rinds into food processor and pulse until finely ground.
2. Place mozzarella into a large microwave-safe bowl.
3. Break cream cheese into small pieces and add them to the bowl. Microwave for 30 seconds, or until both cheeses are melted and can easily be stirred together into a ball.
4. Add ground pork rinds and egg to the cheese mixture.
5. Continue stirring until the mixture forms a ball. If it cools too much and cheese hardens, microwave for 10 more seconds.

6. Separate the dough into four small balls. Place each ball of dough between two sheets of parchment and roll into V4" flat layer.
7. Place tortillas into the air fryer basket in single layer, working in batches if necessary.
8. Adjust the temperature to 400°F and set the timer for 5 minutes.
9. Tortillas will be crispy and firm when fully cooked. Serve immediately.

PER SERVING

Calories: 145 Protein: 10.7 G Fiber: 0.0 G
Net Carbohydrates: 0.8 G Fat: 10.0 G Sodium: 291
Mg Carbohydrates: 0.8 G Sugar: 0.5 G

Garlic Cheese Bread

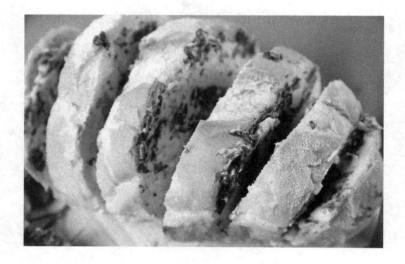

Who would've ever thought it would be so easy to satisfy your Garlic Cheese Bread cravings without an ounce of flour? Here's a keto-friendly appetizer that tastes just like delivery! Take it to the next level by dipping these strips in a low-carb marinara sauce!

- **Hands On Time**: 10 minutes

- **Cook Time**: 10 minutes

Serves 2

Ingredients:

- 1 cup shredded mozzarella cheese

- 1/4 cup grated Parmesan cheese

- 1 large egg

- 1/2 teaspoon garlic powder

Directions

1. Mix all ingredients in a large bowl.
2. Cut a piece of parchment to fit your air fryer basket.
3. Press the mixture into a circle on the parchment and place into the air fryer basket.
4. Adjust the temperature to 350°F and set the timer for 10 minutes. ✓ Serve warm.

PER SERVING

Calories: 258

Protein: 19.2 G Fiber: 0.1 G Net Carbohydrates: 3.6 G Fat: 16.6 G Sodium: 612 Mg Carbohydrates: 3.7 G Sugar: 0.7 G Hidden Carbs

Note

Don't forget that cheese and eggs have carbs. Many nutrition labels round down if the amount is less than 1. An egg, for example, has 0.06 grams of carbs, even though it's often assumed to be carb-free.

Pesto Crackers

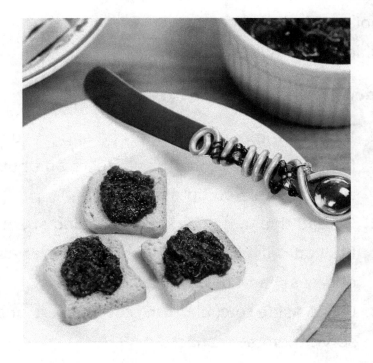

Preparation time: 10 minutes

Cooking time: 17 minutes

Servings: 6

Ingredients:

1/2 teaspoon baking powder
Salt and black pepper to the taste 1 and 1/4 cups
flour

1/4 teaspoon basil, dried

1 garlic clove, minced

2 tablespoons basil pesto

3 tablespoons butter

Directions:

1. In a bowl, mix salt, pepper, baking powder, flour, garlic, cayenne, basil, pesto and butter and stir until you obtain a dough.
2. Spread this dough on a lined baking sheet that fits your air fryer, introduce in the fryer at 325 degrees F and bake for 17 minutes.
3. Leave aside to cool down, cut crackers and serve them as a snack.
   Enjoy!

Nutrition: calories 200, fat 20, fiber 1, carbs 4, protein 7

Apple Chips

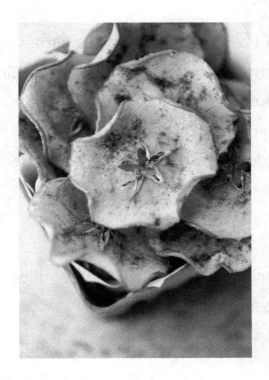

Preparation time: 10 minutes

Cooking time: 10 minutes

Servings: 2

Ingredients:

1 apple, cored and sliced

A pinch of salt

1/2 teaspoon cinnamon powder

1 tablespoon Brown sugar

Directions:

1. In a bowl, mix apple slices with salt, sugar and cinnamon, toss, transfer to your air fryer's basket, cook for 10 minutes at 390 degrees F flipping once.
2. Divide apple chips in bowls and serve as a snack.
Enjoy!

Nutrition: calories 70, fat 0, fiber 4, carbs 3, protein 1

Banana Chips

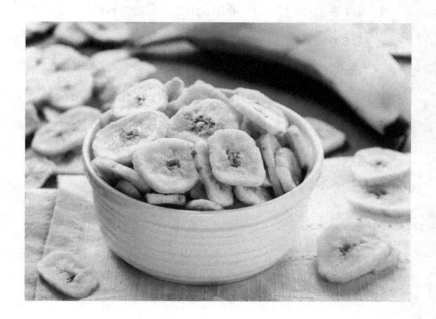

Preparation time: 10 minutes

Cooking time: 15 minutes

Servings: 4

Ingredients:

4 bananas, peeled and sliced A pinch of salt

1/2 teaspoon turmeric powder 1/2 teaspoon chaat masala

1 teaspoon olive oil

Directions:

1. In a bowl, mix banana slices with salt, turmeric, chaat masala and oil, toss and leave aside for 10 minutes.
2. Transfer banana slices to your preheated air fryer at 360 degrees F and cook them for 15 minutes flipping them once.
3. Serve as a snack.

   Enjoy!

Nutrition: calories 121, fat 1, fiber 2, carbs 3, protein 3

Mozzarella Sticks

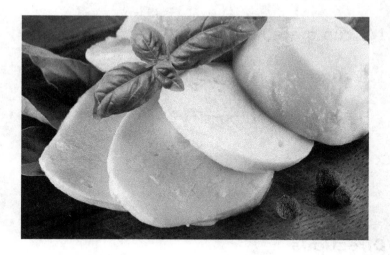

Just like your restaurant favorites, these Mozzarella Sticks are covered in a crispy coating (but this coating is carb-free!) and full of gooey and delicious mozzarella. Pair this with your favorite low- carb marinara sauce, and dig right in! You can even customize it with your favorite kind of cheese for a different flavor profile.

• **Hands On Time**: 1 hour

• **Cook Time**: 10 minutes

Yields 12 sticks (3 per serving)

Ingredients:

6 (1-ounce) mozzarella string cheese sticks

- 1/2 cup grated Parmesan cheese

- 1/2 ounce pork rinds, finely ground

- 1 teaspoon dried parsley

- 2 large eggs

Directions

1. Place mozzarella sticks on a cutting board and cut in half. Freeze 45 minutes or until firm. If freezing overnight, remove frozen sticks after 1 hour and place into airtight zip-top storage bag and place back in freezer for future use.
2. In a large bowl, mix Parmesan, ground pork rinds, and parsley.
3. In a medium bowl, whisk eggs.
4. Dip a frozen mozzarella stick into beaten eggs and then into Parmesan mixture to coat.
5. Repeat with remaining sticks.

6. Place mozzarella sticks into the air fryer basket.

7. Adjust the temperature to 400°F and set the timer for 10 minutes or until golden. Serve warm.

PER SERVING

Calories: 236

Protein: 19.2 G Fiber: 0.0 G

Net Carbohydrates: 4.7 G Fat: 13.8 G

Sodium: 609 Mg Carbohydrates: 4.7 G Sugar: 1.1 G

Bacon-Wrapped Onion Rings

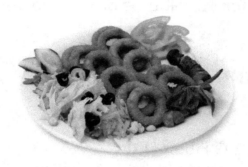

These perfectly crispy onion rings can elevate your game day or take your juicy bunless burger to the next level. A medium onion has around 10 grams of carbs, which can seem high when you're limiting yourself to 20-50 grams of carbs per day. The zero-carb breading increases the fat and protein content for this appetizer, making it an even better keto option, as long as you enjoy in moderation.

• **Hands On Time**: 5 minutes

• **Cook Time**: 10 minutes

Serves 4

Ingredients:

- 1 large onion, peeled

- 1 tablespoon sriracha

- 8 slices sugar-free bacon

Directions

1. Slice onion into 1/4"-thick slices. Brush sriracha over the onion slices.
2. Take two slices of onion and wrap bacon around the rings. Repeat with remaining onion and bacon.
3. Place into the air fryer basket.
4. Adjust the temperature to 350°F and set the timer for 10 minutes.
5. Use tongs to flip the onion rings halfway through the cooking time. When fully cooked, bacon will be crispy. Serve warm.

PER SERVING

Calories: 105 Protein: 7.5 G Fiber: 0.6 G Net Carbohydrates: 3.7 G Fat: 5.9 G Sodium: 401 Mg Carbohydrates: 4.3 G Sugar: 2.3 G

Mini Sweet Pepper Poppers

These crunchy bites are perfectly portioned, poppable peppers to please your palate. This bright and colorful twist on jalapeno poppers comes in bite-sized fun with bold flavor!

- **HandsOn Time**: 15 minutes

- **Cook Time**: 8 minutes

 Yields 16 halves (4 per serving)

Ingredients:

- 8 mini sweet peppers

- 4 ounces full-fat cream cheese, softened

- 4 slices sugar-free bacon, cooked and crumbled

- 1/4 cup shredded pepper jack cheese

Directions

1. Remove the tops from the peppers and slice each one in half lengthwise.
2. Use a small knife to remove seeds and membranes.

3. n a small bowl, mix cream cheese, bacon, and pepper jack.

4. Place 3 teaspoons of the mixture into each sweet pepper and press down smooth. Place into the fryer basket.

5. Adjust the temperature to 400°F and set the timer for 8 minutes. ✓ Serve warm.

PER SERVING

Calories: 176 Protein: 7.4 G
Fiber: 0.9 G
Net Carbohydrates: 2.7 G Fat: 13.4 G Sodium: 309
Mg Carbohydrates: 3.6 G Sugar: 2.2 G

Spicy Spinach Artichoke Dip

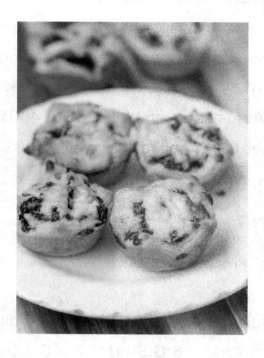

This spicy twist on a classic appetizer pairs cool and creamy with jalapenos for the heavenly appetizer that every party needs! It's right at home on a platter of pork rinds or your favorite low- carb veggies, such as sliced cucumbers or celery sticks.

• **Hands On Time:** 10 minutes

• **Cook Time:** 10 minutes

Serves 6

Ingredients:

- 10 ounces frozen spinach, drained and thawed

- 1 (14-ounce) can artichoke hearts, drained and chopped

- 1/4 cup chopped pickled jalapenos

- 8 ounces full-fat cream cheese, softened

- 1/4 cup full-fat mayonnaise

- 1/4 cup full-fat sour cream

- 1/2 teaspoon garlic powder

- 1/4 cup grated Parmesan cheese

- 1 cup shredded pepper jack cheese

Directions

1. Mix all ingredients in a 4-cup baking bowl. Place into the air fryer basket.

2. Adjust the temperature to 320°F and set the timer for 10 minutes.

3. Remove when brown and bubbling. Serve warm.

PER SERVING

Calories: 226 Protein: 10.0 G Fiber: 3.7 G

Net Carbohydrates: 6.5 G Fat: 15.9 G Sodium: 776

Mg Carbohydrates: 10.2 G Sugar: 3.4 G

Crustless Three-Meat Pizza

Not all pizzas need a crust. And you can achieve crispy pizza perfection from scratch in minutes with this recipe. Even better, you can get creative with toppings to really make this pizza your own. Try topping with an Alfredo sauce and fresh veggies or a low-carb barbecue sauce and grilled chicken!

- **Hands On Time**: 5 minutes
- **Cook Time**: 5 minutes

Serves 1

Ingredients:

- V2 cup shredded mozzarella cheese

- 7 slices pepperoni

- V4 cup cooked ground sausage

- 2 slices sugar-free bacon, cooked and crumbled

- 1 tablespoon grated Parmesan cheese

- 2 tablespoons low- carb, sugar-free pizza sauce, for dipping

---

Directions

1. Cover the bottom of a 6" cake pan with mozzarella.
2. Place pepperoni, sausage, and bacon on top of cheese and sprinkle with Parmesan.
3. Place pan into the air fryer basket.
4. Adjust the temperature to 400°F and set the timer for 5 minutes.
5. Remove when cheese is bubbling and golden.
6. Serve warm with pizza sauce for dipping.

PER SERVING

Calories: 466

Protein: 28.1 G Fiber: 0.5 G

Net Carbohydrates: 4.7 G Fat: 34.0 G

Sodium: 1,446 Mg Carbohydrates: 5.2 G Sugar: 1.6 G

Bacon-Wrapped Brie

Many followers of the keto diet love to snack on cheese. That's because it has minimal carbs and is very convenient. Why not take it to the next level by wrapping the cheese in bacon? After you try this warm wheel of creamy cheese, you'll never want to go back to regular cheese!

- **Hands On Time**: 5 minutes

- Cook Time: 10 minutes

Serves 8

Ingredients:

- 4 slices sugar-free bacon

- 1 (8-ounce) round Brie

Directions

1. Place two slices of bacon to form an X. Place the third slice of bacon horizontally across the center of the X.

2. Place the fourth slice of bacon vertically across the X. It should look like a plus sign (+) on top of an X.
3. Place the Brie in the center of the bacon.
4. Wrap the bacon around the Brie, securing with a few toothpicks.
5. Cut a piece of parchment to fit your air fryer basket and place the bacon-wrapped Brie on top.
6. Place inside the air fryer basket.
7. Adjust the temperature to 400°F and set the timer for 10 minutes.
8. When 3 minutes remain on the timer, carefully flip Brie.
9. When cooked, bacon will be crispy and cheese will be soft and melty. To serve, cut into eight slices.

PER SERVING

Calories: 116 Protein: 7.7 G Fiber: 0.0 G Net Carbohydrates: 0.2 G Fat: 8.9 G Sodium: 259 Mg Carbohydrates: 0.2 G Sugar: 0.1 G

Smoky BBQ Roasted Almonds

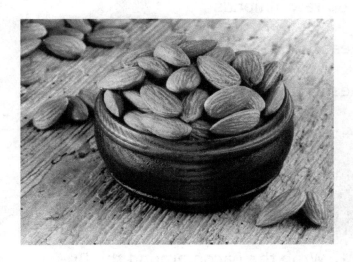

As far as nuts go, almonds are a great low-carb option with plenty of healthy protein instead of carbs. A lot of flavored almonds you might find at your grocery store can be tasty but are usually processed with unnecessary ingredients, like maltodextrin, that can actually raise your blood sugar. This is a clean recipe for a flavorful snack any time of day!

• **Hands On Time**: 5 minutes

• **Cook Time**: 6 minutes Serves 4 (1/4 cup per serving)

Ingredients:

- 1 cup raw almonds

- 2 teaspoons coconut oil

- 1 teaspoon chili powder

- 1/4 teaspoon cumin

- 1/4 teaspoon smoked paprika

- 1/4 teaspoon onion powder

1. Wrap the bacon around the Brie, securing with a few toothpicks.
2. Cut a piece of parchment to fit your air fryer basket and place the bacon-wrapped Brie on top.
3. Place inside the air fryer basket.
4. Adjust the temperature to 400°F and set the timer for 10 minutes.
5. When 3 minutes remain on the timer, carefully flip Brie.
6. When cooked, bacon will be crispy and cheese will be soft and melty. To serve, cut into eight slices.

Directions

1. In a large bowl, toss all ingredients until almonds are evenly coated with oil and spices.
2. Place almonds into the air fryer basket.
3. Adjust the temperature to 320°F and set the timer for 6 minutes.
4. Toss the fryer basket halfway through the cooking time.
5. Allow to cool completely.

PER SERVING

Calories: 182 Protein: 6.2 G

Fiber: 3.3 G

Net Carbohydrates: 3.3 G Fat: 16.3 G Sodium: 19

Mg Carbohydrates: 6.6 G Sugar: 1.1 G

Pork Rind Nachos

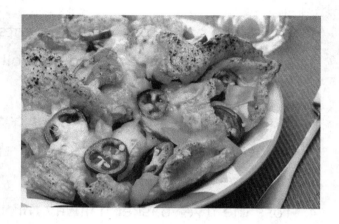

Pork rinds are the ultimate replacement for chips. They're crunchy and flavorful, and best of all, they have zero carbs! Warm and gooey Pork Rind Nachos are a great snack for any time of day, and your air fryer will get the flavors just right!

- **Hands On Time**: 5 minutes

- **Cook Time**: 5 minutes

Serves 2

Ingredients:

- 1 ounce pork rinds

- 4 ounces shredded cooked chicken

- 2 cup shredded Monterey jack cheese

- 4 cup sliced pickled jalapenos

- 4 cup guacamole

- 4 cup full- fat sour cream

Directions

1. Place pork rinds into 6" round baking pan. Cover with shredded chicken and Monterey jack cheese.
2. Place pan into the air fryer basket.
3. Adjust the temperature to 370°F and set the timer for 5 minutes or until cheese is melted.
4. Top with jalapenos, guacamole, and sour cream. Serve immediately.

PER SERVING

Calories: 395 Protein: 30.1 G Fiber: 1.2 G
Net Carbohydrates: 1.8 G Fat: 27.5 G Sodium: 763
Mg Carbohydrates: 3.0 G Sugar: 1.0 G

Mozzarella-Stuffed Meatballs

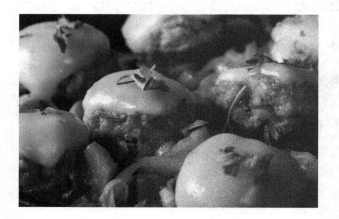

The only thing better than juicy meatballs are juicy meatballs stuffed with gooey, melty cheese! You can enjoy this simple-to- season and easy-to-bake appetizer as is, or pump up the flavor by serving in a low-carb marinara sauce!

• **Hands On Time**: 15 minutes

• **Cook Time**: 15 minutes

Yields 16 meatballs (4 per serving)

Ingredients:

- 1 pound 80/20 ground beef

- 1/4 cup blanched finely ground almond flour

- 1 teaspoon dried parsley

- 1/2 teaspoon garlic powder

- 1/4 teaspoon onion powder

- 1 large egg

- 3 ounces low-moisture, whole-milk mozzarella, cubed

- 1/2 cup low-carb, no-sugar-added pasta sauce

- 1/4 cup grated Parmesan cheese

Directions

1. In a large bowl, add ground beef, almond flour, parsley, garlic powder, onion powder, and egg.
2. Fold ingredients together until fully combined.
3. Form the mixture into 2" balls and use your thumb or a spoon to create an indent in the center of each meatball.

4. Place a cube of cheese in the center and form the ball around it.

5. Place the meatballs into the air fryer, working in batches if necessary.

6. Adjust the temperature to 350°F and set the timer for 15 minutes. Meatballs will be slightly crispy on the outside and fully cooked when at least 180°F internally.

7. When they are finished cooking, toss the meatballs in the sauce and sprinkle with grated Parmesan for serving.

PER SERVING

Calories: 447 Protein: 29.6 G Fiber: 1.8 G
Net Carbohydrates: 3.6 G Fat: 29.7 G Sodium: 509
Mg Carbohydrates: 5.4 G Sugar: 1.6 G

Ranch Roasted Almonds

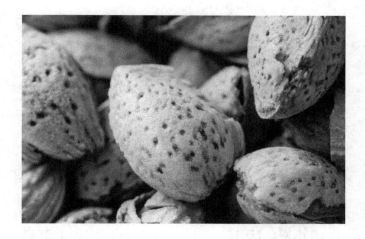

Roasted almonds are low in carbs, but high in fiber and fats. They have a crunch that's hard to come by in low-carb foods and will satisfy your snacking urges. The only potential problem is their bland flavor, which this recipe eliminates completely!

• **Hands On Time**: 5 minutes

• **Cook Time**: 6 minutes

 Yields 2 cups (V4 cup per serving)

Ingredients:

- 2 cups raw almonds

- 2 tablespoons unsalted butter, melted

- 2 (1-ounce) ranch dressing mix packet

Directions

1. In a large bowl, toss almonds in butter to evenly coat.
2. Sprinkle ranch mix over almonds and toss. Place almonds into the air fryer basket.
3. Adjust the temperature to 320°F and set the timer for 6 minutes.
4. Shake the basket two or three times during cooking.
5. Let cool at least 20 minutes. Almonds will be soft but become crunchier during cooling.
6. Store in an airtight container up to 3 days.

PER SERVING

Calories: 190

Protein: 6.0 G Fiber: 3.0 G

Net Carbohydrates: 4.0 G Fat: 16.7 G

Coconut Chicken Bites

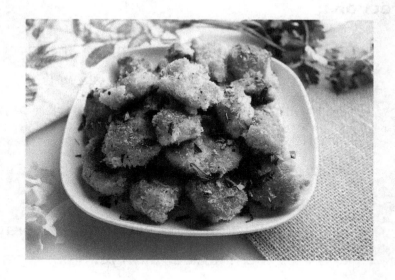

Preparation time: 10 minutes

Cooking time: 13 minutes

Servings: 4

Ingredients:

2 teaspoons garlic powder

2 eggs

3/4 cup panko bread crumbs 3/4 cup coconut,
shredded Cooking spray

8 chicken tenders

Salt and black pepper to the taste

Directions:

1. In a bowl, mix eggs with salt, pepper and garlic powder and whisk well.
2. In another bowl, mix coconut with panko and stir well.
3. Dip chicken tenders in eggs mix and then coat in coconut one well.
4. Spray chicken bites with cooking spray, place them in your air fryer's basket and cook them at 350 degrees F for 10 minutes.
5. Arrange them on a platter and serve as an appetizer. Enjoy!

Nutrition: calories 252, fat 4, fiber 2, carbs 14, protein 24

Buffalo Cauliflower Snack

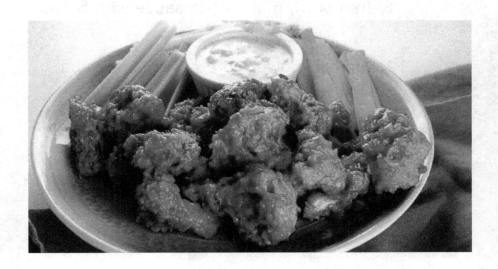

Preparation time: 10 minutes

Cooking time: 15 minutes

Servings: 4

Ingredients:

4 cups cauliflower florets 1 cup panko bread crumbs

1/4 cup butter, melted

1/4 cup buffalo sauce Mayonnaise for serving

Directions:

1. In a bowl, mix buffalo sauce with butter and whisk well.
2. Dip cauliflower florets in this mix and coat them in panko bread crumbs.
3. Place them in your air fryer's basket and cook at 350 degrees F for 15 minutes.
4. Arrange them on a platter and serve with mayo on the side. Enjoy!

Nutrition: calories 241, fat 4, fiber 7, carbs 8, protein 4

Banana Snack

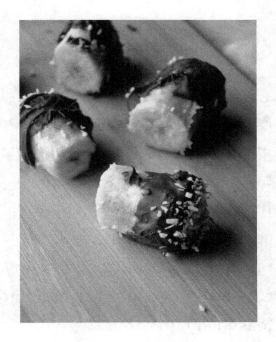

Preparation time: 10 minutes

Cooking time: 5 minutes

Servings: 8

Ingredients:

16 baking cups crust
1/4 cup peanut butter
3/4 cup chocolate chips

1 banana, peeled and sliced into 16 pieces 1 tablespoon vegetable oil

Directions:

1. Put chocolate chips in a small pot, heat up over low heat, stir until it melts and take off heat.
2. In a bowl, mix peanut butter with coconut oil and whisk well.
3. Spoon 1 teaspoon chocolate mix in a cup, add 1 banana slice and top with 1 teaspoon butter mix
4. Repeat with the rest of the cups, place them all into a dish that fits your air fryer, cook at 320 degrees F for 5 minutes, transfer to a freezer and keep there until you serve them as a snack. Enjoy!

Nutrition: calories 70, fat 4, fiber 1, carbs 10, protein 1

Potato Spread

Preparation time: 10 minutes

Cooking time: 10 minutes

Servings: 10

Ingredients:

19 ounces canned garbanzo beans, drained

1 cup sweet potatoes, peeled and chopped 1/4 cup tahini

2 tablespoons lemon juice 1 tablespoon olive oil
5 garlic cloves, minced
1/2 teaspoon cumin, ground 2 tablespoons water

A pinch of salt and white pepper

Directions:

1. Put potatoes in your air fryer's basket, cook them at 360 degrees F for 15 minutes, cool them down, peel, put them in your food processor and pulse well. basket,

2. Add sesame paste, garlic, beans, lemon juice, cumin, water and oil and pulse really well.
3. Add salt and pepper, pulse again, divide into bowls and serve.

Enjoy!

Nutrition: calories 200, fat 3, fiber 10, carbs 20, protein 11

Mexican Apple Snack

Preparation time: 10 minutes

Cooking time: 5 minutes

Servings: 4

Ingredients:

3 big apples, cored, peeled and cubed 2 teaspoons
lemon juice
1/4 cup pecans, chopped
1/2 cup dark chocolate chips

1/2 cup clean caramel sauce

Directions:

1. In a bowl, mix apples with lemon juice,
   stir and transfer to a pan that fits your
   air fryer.
2. Add chocolate chips, pecans, drizzle the
   caramel sauce, toss, introduce in your
   air fryer and cook at 320 degrees F for 5
   minutes.

3. Toss gently, divide into small bowls and serve right away as a snack.
Enjoy!

Nutrition: calories 200, fat 4, fiber 3, carbs 20, protein 3

Shrimp Muffins

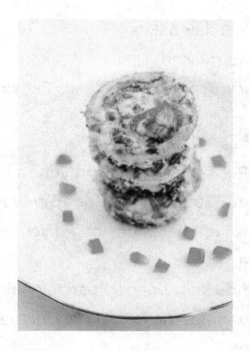

Preparation time: 10 minutes

Cooking time: 26 minutes

Servings: 6

Ingredients:

1 spaghetti squash, peeled and halved

2 tablespoons mayonnaise

1 cup mozzarella, shredded

8 ounces shrimp, peeled, cooked and chopped 1 and 1/2 cups panko

1 teaspoon parsley flakes

1 garlic clove, minced

Salt and black pepper to the taste Cooking spray

Directions:

1. Put squash halves in your air fryer, cook at 350 degrees F for 16 minutes, leave aside to cool down and scrape flesh into a bowl.
2. Add salt, pepper, parsley flakes, panko, shrimp, mayo and mozzarella and stir well.
3. Spray a muffin tray that fits your air fryer with cooking spray and divide squash and shrimp mix in each cup.
4. Introduce in the fryer and cook at 360 degrees F for 10 minutes. Arrange muffins on a platter and serve as a snack. Enjoy!

   Nutrition: calories 60, fat 2, fiber 0.4, carbs 4, protein 4

Zucchini Cakes

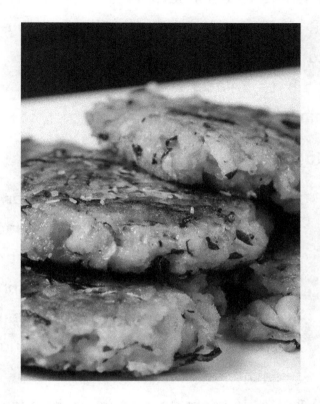

Preparation time: 10 minutes

Cooking time: 12 minutes

Servings: 12

Ingredients:

Cooking spray

1/2 cup dill, chopped

1 egg

1/2 cup whole wheat flour

Salt and black pepper to the taste 1 yellow onion, chopped

2 garlic cloves, minced

3 zucchinis, grated

Directions:

1. In a bowl, mix zucchinis with garlic, onion, flour, salt, pepper, egg and dill, stir well, shape small patties out of this mix, spray them with cooking spray, place them in your air fryer's basket.
2. Cook at 370 degrees F for 6 minutes on each side.
3. Serve them as a snack right away. Enjoy!

Nutrition: calories 60, fat 1, fiber 2, carbs 6, protein 2

Cauliflower Bars

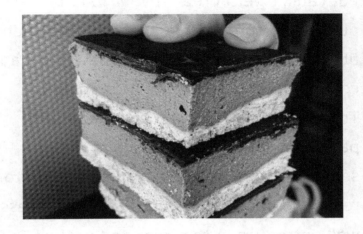

Preparation time: 10 minutes

Cooking time: 25 minutes

Servings: 12

Ingredients:

1 big cauliflower head,

florets separated 1/2 cup mozzarella, shredded

1/4 cup egg whites

1 teaspoon Italian seasoning

Salt and black pepper to the taste

Directions:

1. Put cauliflower florets in your food processor, pulse well, spread on a lined baking sheet that fits your air fryer, introduce in the fryer and cook at 360 degrees F for 10 minutes.
2. Transfer cauliflower to a bowl, add salt, pepper, cheese, egg whites and Italian seasoning, stir really well, spread this into a rectangle pan that fits your air fryer, press well, introduce in the fryer and cook at 360 degrees F for 15 minutes more.
3. Cut into 12 bars, arrange them on a platter and serve as a snack Enjoy!

Nutrition: calories 50, fat 1, fiber 2, carbs 3, protein 3

Pumpkin Muffins

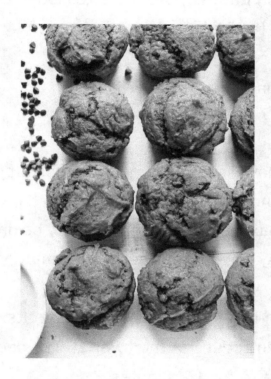

Preparation time: 10 minutes

Cooking time: 15 minutes

Servings: 18

Ingredients:

1/4 cup butter

3/4 cup pumpkin puree

2 tablespoons flaxseed meal 1/4 cup flour

1/2 cup sugar

1/2 teaspoon nutmeg, ground 1 teaspoon cinnamon powder 1/2 teaspoon baking soda

1 egg

1/2 teaspoon baking powder

Directions:

1. In a bowl, mix butter with pumpkin puree and egg and blend well.
2. Add flaxseed meal, flour, sugar, baking soda, baking powder, nutmeg and cinnamon and stir well.
3. Spoon this into a muffin pan that fits your fryer introduce in the fryer at 350 degrees F and bake for 15 minutes.
4. Serve muffins cold as a snack.

   Enjoy!

   Nutrition: calories 50, fat 3, fiber 1, carbs 2, protein 2

Zucchini Chips

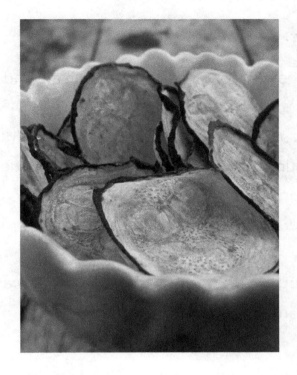

Preparation time: 10 minutes

Cooking time: 1 hour

Servings: 6

Ingredients:

3 zucchinis, thinly sliced

Salt and black pepper to the taste 2 tablespoons

olive oil

2 tablespoons balsamic vinegar

Directions:

1. In a bowl, mix oil with vinegar, salt and pepper and whisk well.
2. Add zucchini slices, toss to coat well, introduce in your air fryer and cook at 200 degrees F for 1 hour.
3. Serve zucchini chips cold as a snack. Enjoy!

   Nutrition: calories 40, fat 3, fiber 7, carbs 3, protein 7

Beef Jerky Snack

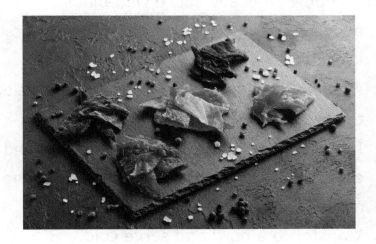

Preparation time: 2 hours

Cooking time: 1 hour and 30 minutes

Servings: 6

 Ingredients:

2 cups soy sauce

1/2 cup Worcestershire sauce

2 tablespoons black peppercorns 2 tablespoons
black pepper

2 pounds beef round, sliced

Directions:

1. In a bowl, mix soy sauce with black peppercorns, black pepper and Worcestershire sauce and whisk well.
2. Add beef slices, toss to coat and leave aside in the fridge for 6 hours.
3. Introduce beef rounds in your air fryer and cook them at 370 degrees F for 1 hour and 30 minutes.
4. Transfer to a bowl and serve cold.
   Enjoy!

Nutrition: calories 300, fat 12, fiber 4, carbs 3, protein 8

Honey Party Wings

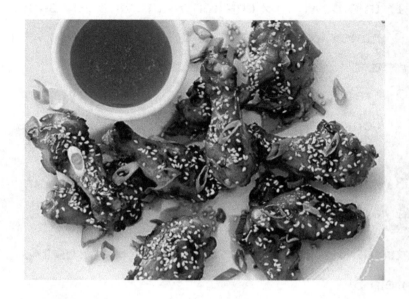

Preparation time: 1 hour and 10 minutes

Cooking time: 12 minutes

Servings:8

Ingredients:

16 chicken wings, halved

2 tablespoons soy sauce

2 tablespoons honey

Salt and black pepper to the taste 2 tablespoons

lime juice

Directions:

1. In a bowl, mix chicken wings with soy sauce, honey, salt, pepper and lime juice, toss well and keep in the fridge for 1 hour.
2. Transfer chicken wings to your air fryer and cook them at 360 degrees F for 12 minutes, flipping them halfway.
3. Arrange them on a platter and serve as an appetizer. Enjoy!

Nutrition: calories 211, fat 4, fiber 7, carbs 14, protein 3

Salmon Party Patties

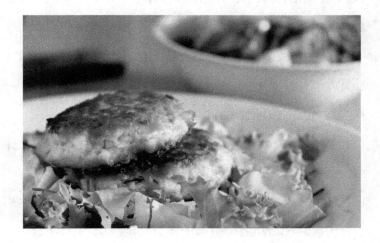

Preparation time: 10 minutes

Cooking time: 22 minutes

Servings: 4

Ingredients:

3 big potatoes, boiled, drained and mashed 1 big
salmon fillet, skinless, boneless
2 tablespoons parsley, chopped
2 tablespoon dill, chopped

Salt and black pepper to the taste 1 egg
2 tablespoons bread crumbs Cooking spray

Directions:

1. Place salmon in your air fryer's basket and cook for 10 minutes at 360 degrees F.
2. Transfer salmon to a cutting board, cool it down, flake it and put it in a bowl.
3. Add mashed potatoes, salt, pepper, dill, parsley, egg and bread crumbs, stir well and shape 8 patties out of this mix.
4. Place salmon patties in your air fryer's basket, spry them with cooking oil, cook at 360 degrees F for 12 minutes, flipping them halfway, transfer them to a platter and serve as an appetizer. Enjoy!

Nutrition: calories 231, fat 3, fiber 7, carbs 14, protein 4

Spring Rolls

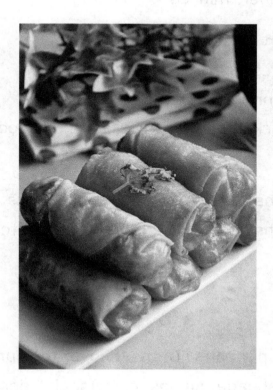

Preparation time: 10 minutes

Cooking time: 25 minutes

 Servings: 8

Ingredients:

2 cups green cabbage, shredded 2 yellow onions, chopped

1 carrot, grated

1/2 chili pepper, minced

1 tablespoon ginger, grated

3 garlic cloves, minced

1 teaspoon brown sugar

Salt and black pepper to the taste 1 teaspoon soy sauce

2 tablespoons olive oil 10 spring roll sheets

2 tablespoons corn flour 2 tablespoons water

Directions:

1. Heat up a pan with the oil over medium heat, add cabbage, onions, carrots, chili pepper, ginger, garlic, sugar, salt, pepper and soy sauce, stir well, cook for 2-3 minutes, take off heat and cool down.

2. Cut spring roll sheets in squares, divide cabbage mix on each and roll them.
   In a bowl, mix corn flour with water, stir well and seal spring rolls with this mix.

3. Place spring rolls in your air fryer's basket and cook them at 360 degrees F for 10 minutes.
4. Flip roll and cook them for 10 minutes more.
5. Arrange on a platter and serve them as an appetizer. Enjoy!

Nutrition: calories 214, fat 4, fiber 4, carbs 12, protein 4

Crispy Radish Chips

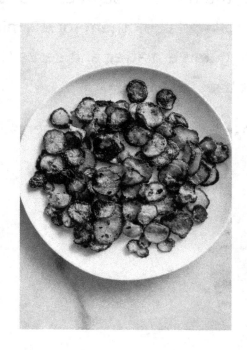

Preparation time: 10 minutes

Cooking time: 10 minutes

Servings: 4

Ingredients:

Cooking spray

15 radishes, sliced

Salt and black pepper to the taste 1 tablespoon chives, chopped

Directions:

1. Arrange radish slices in your air fryer's basket, spray them with cooking oil, season with salt and black pepper to the taste.
2. Cook them at 350 degrees F for 10 minutes, flipping them halfway.
3. Transfer to bowls and serve with chives sprinkled on top.

   Enjoy!

   Nutrition: calories 80, fat 1, fiber 1, carbs 1, protein 1

Crab Sticks

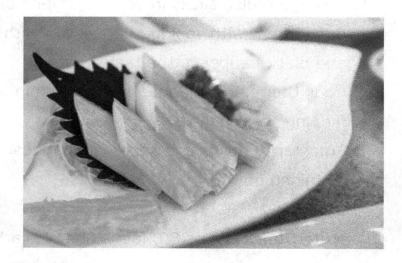

Preparation time: 10 minutes

Cooking time: 12 minutes

Servings: 4

Ingredients:

10 crabsticks, halved

2 teaspoons sesame oil

2 teaspoons Cajun seasoning

Directions:

1. Put crab sticks in a bowl, add sesame oil and Cajun seasoning, toss, transfer them to your

air fryer's basket and cook at 350 degrees F
for 12 minutes.

2. Arrange on a platter and serve as an
appetizer.

Enjoy!

Nutrition: calories 110, fat 0, fiber 1, carbs 4,
protein 2

Air Fried Dill Pickles

Preparation time: 10 minutes

Cooking time: 5 minutes

Servings: 4

Ingredients:

16 ounces jarred dill pickles, cut into wedges and pat dried 1/2 cup white flour

1 egg

1/4 cup milk

1/2 teaspoon garlic powder 1/2 teaspoon sweet paprika Cooking spray

1/4 cup ranch sauce

Directions:

1. In a bowl, combine milk with egg and whisk well.
2. In a second bowl, mix flour with salt, garlic powder and paprika and stir as well
3. Dip pickles in flour, then in egg mix and again in flour and place them in your air fryer.

4. Grease them with cooking spray, cook pickle wedges at 400 degrees F for 5 minutes, transfer to a bowl and serve with ranch sauce on the side.

Enjoy!

Nutrition: calories 109, fat 2, fiber 2, carbs 10, protein 4

Chickpeas Snack

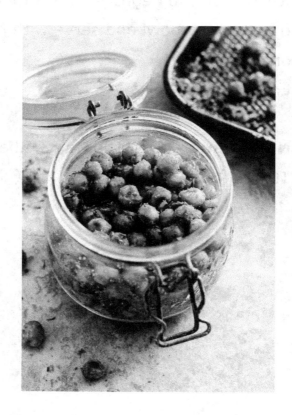

Preparation time: 10 minutes

Cooking time: 10 minutes

Servings: 4

Ingredients:

15 ounces canned chickpeas, drained 1/2 teaspoon cumin, ground

1 tablespoon olive oil

1 teaspoon smoked paprika

Salt and black pepper to the taste

Directions:

1. In a bowl, mix chickpeas with oil, cumin, paprika, salt and pepper, toss to coat.
2. Place them in your fryer's basket and cook at 390 degrees F for 10 minutes.
3. Divide into bowls and serve as a snack.

Enjoy!

Nutrition: calories 140, fat 1, fiber 6, carbs 20, protein 6

Sausage Balls

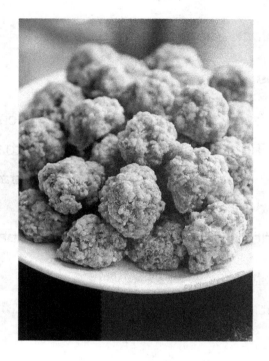

Preparation time: 10 minutes

Cooking time: 15 minutes

Servings: 9

Ingredients:

4 ounces sausage meat, ground Salt and black
pepper to the taste 1 teaspoon sage
1/2 teaspoon garlic, minced

1 small onion, chopped

3 tablespoons breadcrumbs

Directions:

1. In a bowl, mix sausage with salt, pepper, sage, garlic, onion and breadcrumbs,
2. Stir well and shape small balls out of this mix.
3. Put them in your air fryer's basket,
4. Cook at 360 degrees F for 15 minutes.
5. Divide into bowls and serve as a snack.

Enjoy!

Nutrition: calories 130, fat 7, fiber 1, carbs 13, protein 4

Chicken Dip

Preparation time: 10 minutes

Cooking time: 25 minutes

Servings: 10

Ingredients:

3 tablespoons butter, melted

1 cup yogurt

12 ounces cream cheese

2 cups chicken meat, cooked and shredded 2 teaspoons curry powder

4 scallions, chopped

6 ounces Monterey jack cheese, grated 1/3 cup raisins

1/4 cup cilantro, chopped

1/2 cup almonds, sliced

Salt and black pepper to the taste

1/2 cup chutney

Directions:

1. In a bowl mix cream cheese with yogurt and whisk using your mixer.

2. Add curry powder, scallions, chicken meat, raisins, cheese, cilantro, salt and pepper and stir everything.
3. Spread this into a baking dish that fist your air fryer.
4. Sprinkle almonds on top, place in your air fryer, bake at 300 degrees for 25 minutes,
5. Divide into bowls, top with chutney and serve as an appetizer.

   Enjoy!

Nutrition: calories 240, fat 10, fiber 2, carbs 24, protein 12

Sweet Popcorn

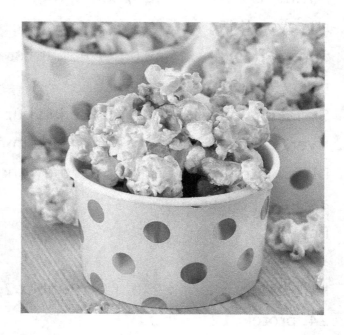

Preparation time: 5 minutes

Cooking time: 10 minutes

Servings: 4

Ingredients:

2 tablespoons corn kernels 2 and 1/2 tablespoons butter 2 ounces brown sugar

Directions:

1. Put corn kernels in your air fryer's pan, cook at 400 degrees F for 6 minutes, transfer them to a tray.
2. Spread and leave aside for now.
3. Heat up a pan over low heat, add butter, melt it, add sugar and stir until it dissolves.
4. Add popcorn, toss to coat, take off heat and spread on the tray again.
5. Cool down, divide into bowls and serve as a snack. Enjoy!

   Nutrition: calories 70, fat 0.2, fiber 0, carbs 1, protein 1

Bread Sticks

Preparation time: 10 minutes

Cooking time: 10 minutes

Servings: 2

Ingredients:

4 bread slices, each cut into 4 sticks 2 eggs

1/4 cup milk

1 teaspoon cinnamon powder

1 tablespoon honey

1/4 cup brown sugar A pinch of nutmeg

Directions:

1. In a bowl, mix eggs with milk, brown sugar, cinnamon, nutmeg and honey and whisk well.
2. Dip bread sticks in this mix, place them in your air fryer's basket and cook at 360 degrees F for 10 minutes.
3. Divide bread sticks into bowls and serve as a snack. Enjoy!
   Nutrition: calories 140, fat 1, fiber 4, carbs 8, protein 4

Crispy Shrimp

Preparation time: 10 minutes

Cooking time: 5 minutes

Servings: 4

Ingredients:

12 big shrimp, deveined and peeled 2 egg whites
1 cup coconut, shredded
1 cup panko bread crumbs 1 cup white flour, Salt
and black pepper to the taste

Directions:

1. In a bowl, mix panko with coconut and stir.
   Put flour, salt and pepper in a second bowl
   and whisk egg whites in a third one.
2. Dip shrimp in flour, egg whites mix and
   coconut, place them all in your air fryer's
   basket, cook at 350 degrees F for 10 minutes
   flipping halfway.
3. Arrange on a platter and serve as an
   appetizer. Enjoy!
   Nutrition: calories 140, fat 4, fiber 0, carbs 3,
   protein 4

Cajun Shrimp Appetizer

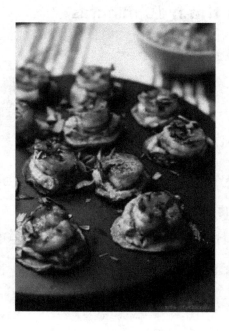

Preparation time: 10 minutes

Cooking time: 5 minutes

Servings: 2

Ingredients:

20 tiger shrimp, peeled and deveined Salt and black
pepper to the taste

1/2 teaspoon old bay seasoning

1 tablespoon olive oil

1/4 teaspoon smoked paprika

Directions:

1. In a bowl, mix shrimp with oil, salt, pepper, old bay seasoning and paprika and toss to coat.
2. Place shrimp in your air fryer's basket and cook at 390 degrees F for 5 minutes. Arrange them on a platter and serve as an appetizer. Enjoy!

Nutrition: calories 162, fat 6, fiber 4, carbs 8, protein 14

Crispy Fish Sticks

Preparation time: 10 minutes

Cooking time: 12 minutes

Servings: 2

Ingredients:

4 ounces bread crumbs

4 tablespoons olive oil

1 egg, whisked

4 white fish filets, boneless, skinless and cut into medium sticks Salt and black pepper to the taste

Directions:

1. In a bowl, mix bread crumbs with oil and stir well.
2. Put egg in a second bowl, add salt and pepper and whisk well.
3. Dip fish stick in egg and them in bread crumb mix, place them in your air fryer's basket and cook at 360 degrees F for 12 minutes.

4. Arrange fish sticks on a platter and serve as an appetizer.

Enjoy!

Nutrition: calories 160, fat 3, fiber 5, carbs 12, protein 3

Fish Nuggets

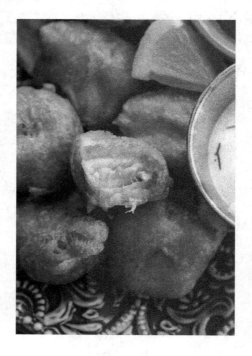

Preparation time: 10 minutes

Cooking time: 12 minutes

Servings: 4

Ingredients:

28 ounces fish fillets, skinless and cut into medium pieces Salt and black pepper to the taste

5 tablespoons flour
1 egg, whisked

5 tablespoons water

3 ounces panko bread crumbs 1 tablespoon garlic powder 1 tablespoon smoked paprika

4 tablespoons homemade mayonnaise Lemon juice from 1/2 lemon

1 teaspoon dill, dried Cooking spray

Directions:

1. In a bowl, mix flour with water and stir well. Add egg, salt and pepper and whisk well. In a second bowl, mix panko with garlic powder and paprika and stir well.
2. Dip fish pieces in flour and egg mix and then in panko mix, place them in your air fryer's basket, spray them with cooking oil and cook at 400 degrees F for 12 minutes.
3. Meanwhile, in a bowl mix mayo with dill and lemon juice and whisk well.

Arrange fish nuggets on a platter and serve with dill mayo on the side. Enjoy!

Nutrition: calories 332, fat 12, fiber 6, carbs 17, protein 15

Shrimp and Chestnut Rolls

Preparation time: 10 minutes

Cooking time: 15 minutes

Servings: 4

Ingredients:

1/2 pound already cooked shrimp, chopped 8 ounces water chestnuts, chopped

1/2 pounds shiitake mushrooms, chopped 2 cups cabbage, chopped

2 tablespoons olive oil

1 garlic clove, minced

1 teaspoon ginger, grated

3 scallions, chopped

Salt and black pepper to the taste 1 tablespoon water

1 egg yolk

6 spring roll wrappers

Directions:

1. Heat up a pan with the oil over medium high heat, add cabbage, shrimp, chestnuts, mushrooms, garlic, ginger, scallions, salt and pepper, stir and cook for 2 minutes.
2. In a bowl, mix egg with water and stir well.
3. Arrange roll wrappers on a working surface, divide shrimp and veggie mix on them, seal edges with egg wash, place them all in your air fryer's basket, cook at 360 degrees F for 15 minutes, transfer to a platter and serve as an appetizer. Enjoy!

Nutrition: calories 140, fat 3, fiber 1, carbs 12, protein 3

Seafood Appetizer

Preparation time: 10 minutes

Cooking time: 25 minutes

Servings: 4

Ingredients:

1/2 cup yellow onion, chopped

1 cup green bell pepper, chopped

1 cup celery, chopped

1 cup baby shrimp, peeled and deveined 1 cup

crabmeat, flaked

1 cup homemade mayonnaise

1 teaspoon Worcestershire sauce

Salt and black pepper to the taste

2 tablespoons bread crumbs

1 tablespoon butter

1 teaspoon sweet paprika

Directions:

1. In a bowl, mix shrimp with crab meat, bell
   pepper, onion, mayo, celery, salt and pepper
   and stir.

2. Add Worcestershire sauce, stir again and pour everything into a baking dish that fits your air fryer.
3. Sprinkle bread crumbs and add butter, introduce in your air fryer and cook at 320 degrees F for 25 minutes, shaking halfway.
4. Divide into bowl and serve with paprika sprinkled on top as an appetizer.
   Enjoy!
   Nutrition: calories 200, fat 1, fiber 2, carbs 5, protein 1

Salmon Meatballs

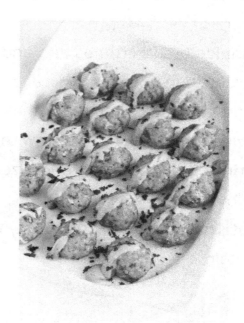

Preparation time: 10 minutes

Cooking time: 12 minutes

Servings: 4

Ingredients:

3 tablespoons cilantro, minced
1 pound salmon, skinless and chopped 1 small
yellow onion, chopped
1 egg white

Salt and black pepper to the taste

2 garlic cloves, minced

1/2 teaspoon paprika

1/4 cup panko

1/2 teaspoon oregano, ground

Cooking spray

Directions:

1. In your food processor, mix salmon with onion, cilantro, egg white, garlic cloves, salt, pepper, paprika and oregano and stir well.
2. Add panko, blend again and shape meatballs from this mix using your palms.
3. Place them in your air fryer's basket, spray them with cooking spray and cook at 320 degrees F for 12 minutes shaking the fryer halfway.
4. Arrange meatballs on a platter and serve them as an appetizer.
   Enjoy!
   Nutrition: calories 289, fat 12, fiber 3, carbs 22, protein 23

Easy Chicken Wings

Preparation time: 10 minutes

Cooking time: 1 hours

Servings: 2

Ingredients:

16 pieces chicken wings

Salt and black pepper to the taste 1/4 cup butter

3/4 cup potato starch

1/4 cup honey

4 tablespoons garlic, minced

Directions:

1. In a bowl, mix chicken wings with salt, pepper and potato starch, toss well, transfer to your air fryer's basket, cook them at 380 degrees F for 25 minutes and at 400 degrees F for 5 minutes more.
2. Meanwhile, heat up a pan with the butter over medium high heat, melt it, add garlic, stir, cook for 5 minutes and then mix with salt, pepper and honey.

3. Whisk well, cook over medium heat for 20 minutes and take off heat.
4. Arrange chicken wings on a platter, drizzle honey sauce all over and serve as an appetizer.

Enjoy!

Nutrition: calories 244, fat 7, fiber 3, carbs 19, protein 8

Chicken Breast Rolls

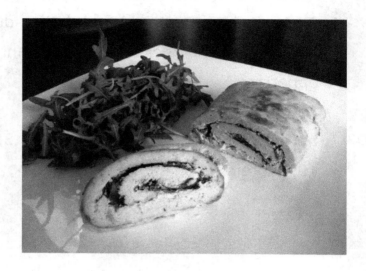

Preparation time: 10 minutes

Cooking time: 22 minutes

Servings: 4

Ingredients:

2 cups baby spinach

4 chicken breasts, boneless and skinless 1 cup sun dried tomatoes, chopped

Salt and black pepper to the taste

1 and 1/2 tablespoons Italian seasoning

4 mozzarella slices

A drizzle of olive oil

Directions:

1. Flatten chicken breasts using a meat tenderizer, divide tomatoes, mozzarella and spinach, season with salt, pepper and Italian seasoning, roll and seal them.
2. Place them in your air fryer's basket, drizzle some oil over them and cook at 375 degrees F for 17 minutes, flipping once.
3. Arrange chicken rolls on a platter and serve them as an appetizer.
   Enjoy!

Nutrition: calories 300, fat 1, fiber 4, carbs 7, protein 10

Crispy Chicken Breast Sticks

Preparation time: 10 minutes

Cooking time: 16 minutes

Servings: 4

Ingredients:

3/4 cup white flour

1 pound chicken breast, skinless, boneless and cut into medium sticks 1 teaspoon sweet paprika

1 cup panko bread crumbs

1 egg, whisked

Salt and black pepper to the taste

1/2 tablespoon olive oil

Zest from 1 lemon, grated

Directions:

1. In a bowl, mix paprika with flour, salt, pepper and lemon zest and stir.
2. Put whisked egg in another bowl and the panko breadcrumbs in a third one.
3. Dredge chicken pieces in flour, egg and panko and place them in your lined air fryer's basket,

drizzle the oil over them, cook at 400 degrees F for 8 minutes, flip and cook for 8 more minutes.

4. Arrange them on a platter and serve as a snack.

   Enjoy!

Nutrition: calories 254, fat 4, fiber 7, carbs 20, protein 22

Beef Roll s

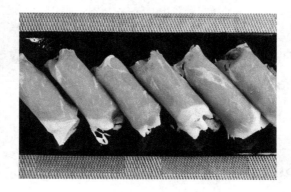

Preparation time: 10 minutes

Cooking time: 14 minutes

Servings: 4

Ingredients:

2 pounds beef steak, opened and flattened with a meat tenderizer Salt and black pepper to the taste

1 cup baby spinach
3 ounces red bell pepper, roasted and chopped 6 slices provolone cheese
3 tablespoons pesto

Directions:

1. Arrange flattened beef steak on a cutting board, spread pesto all over, add cheese in a single layer, add bell peppers, spinach, salt and pepper to the taste.
2. Roll your steak, secure with toothpicks, season again with salt and pepper, place roll in your air fryer's basket and cook at 400 degrees F for 14 minutes, rotating roll halfway.
3. Leave aside to cool down, cut into 2 inch smaller rolls, arrange on a platter and serve them as an appetizer.

Enjoy!

Nutrition: calories 230, fat 1, fiber 3, carbs 12, protein 10

Greek Lamb Meatballs

Preparation time: 10 minutes

Cooking time: 8 minutes

Servings: 10

 Ingredients:

4 ounces lamb meat, minced

Salt and black pepper to the taste

1 slice of bread, toasted and crumbled 2

tablespoons feta cheese, crumbled 1/2 tablespoon

lemon peel, grated

1 tablespoon oregano, chopped

Directions:

In a bowl, combine meat with bread crumbs, salt, pepper, feta, oregano and lemon peel, stir well, shape 10 meatballs and place them in you air fryer.

Cook at 400 degrees F for 8 minutes, arrange them on a platter and serve as an appetizer.

Enjoy!

Nutrition: calories 234, fat 12, fiber 2, carbs 20, protein 30

Empanadas

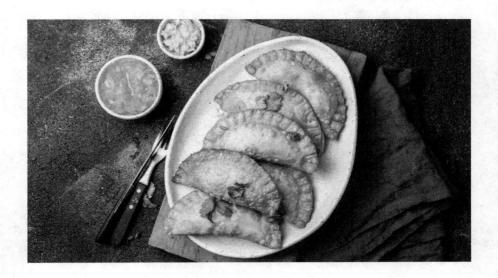

Preparation time: 10 minutes

Cooking time: 25 minutes

Servings: 4

Ingredients: 1 package empanada shells

1 tablespoon olive oil

1 pound beef meat, ground

1 yellow onion, chopped

Salt and black pepper to the taste 2 garlic cloves,

minced 1/2 teaspoon cumin, ground

1/4 cup tomato salsa

1 egg yolk whisked with 1 tablespoon water 1 green bell pepper, chopped

Directions:

1. Heat up a pan with the oil over medium high heat, add beef and brown on all sides.
2. Add onion, garlic, salt, pepper, bell pepper and tomato salsa, stir and cook for 15 minutes.
3. Divide cooked meat in empanada shells, brush them with egg wash and seal.
4. Place them in your air fryer's steamer basket and cook at 350 degrees F for 10 minutes.
5. Arrange on a platter and serve as an appetizer. Enjoy!

Nutrition: calories 274, fat 17, fiber 14, carbs 20, protein 7

CPSIA information can be obtained
at www.ICGtesting.com
Printed in the USA
LVHW081550250421
685458LV00009B/484